STRESS AND ANXIETY:

30 WAYS TO GET RID OF THEM FOR GOOD

By Isabelle Poirier

STRESS AND ANXIETY: 30 WAYS TO GET RID OF THEM FOR GOOD

First Edition: July 2016

TABLE OF CONTENTS

Who am I?

First of all, I want to thank you for buying this book. I promise you it is the first step to your feeling better.

But I know you are wondering who this Isabelle Poirier is? A doctor? A psychiatrist? A psychologist? No, no and no. I am simply a woman in her young thirties who have been living with stress and anxiety for more than twenty years. I can imagine you right now, ready to close this book... Please wait! And answer the following question: who is better suited to tell you what *really works* for controlling your stress and anxiety? A health professional who never suffered from it? Or a person who have been living for many years with that condition and have learned to master it?

Far from me the idea of telling you that all health professional are not equipped adequately to help you. Some of them are helpful. I had the opportunity to meet excellent ones. However, it was not the majority of them, and it did delay me from receiving adequate support for my symptoms. It took me several years to understand what was working and what was not. Today, I never felt much better in my entire life. And I want to share my knowledge with every stressed or anxious person out there. You are not alone, and there are solutions.

In this book, I have listed and explained the 30 ways that helped me regain control over my life. Those 30 ways naturally divided themselves into five categories to work on: Body, Mind, Heart, Soul, and Action. Maybe you won't need all of those pieces of advice. Perhaps just a handful of them will be sufficient for you. Either way, it's okay. All I'm asking you is to keep an open mind.

Finally, you will notice that this book is a short one. Why? Didn't I have enough material to make a 200-and-something pages book? On the contrary. I could talk about this subject for hours even to the point of boring you with it. But I know how difficult it is to take the first step toward a stress and anxiety free life. That is why I wanted to keep this book on the short side. It is concise and straight to the point. And this is what you need right now.

That being said, I really hope this book helps YOU and that you enjoy it.

Isabelle Poirier

P.S. I invite you to check my website or to follow me on my various social media accounts. Do not hesitate to contact me and ask me questions. I will be happy to hear from you.

www.isapoirier.com

www.facebook.com/isapoirier2016

www.twitter.com/isapoirier2016

www.instagram.com/isapoirier2016

www.pinterest.com/isapoirier2016

The price of stress and anxiety

Stress and anxiety (or S/A) are two simple words but very dangerous ones. I see them as a two-headed monster that lurks in every crack of doubt it can find. Maybe you are suffering from one without having the other but in my experience, they come as a package deal, and they share many of the same symptoms, so that's why I am addressing both of them in the same book.

Stress usually comes from external events or situations (like a deadline at work or bills to pay) which cause frustration and nervousness. Anxiety, on the other hand, originates from the fear and worry that we feel. And they can both link very easily. For example, you have an approaching deadline at work, but you have no idea how you are going to make it in time. That causes you frustration and nervousness (*"Why am I not able to achieve this? What is my boss going to say?"*) which then brings you fear and worry (*"Maybe my boss will be so pissed that he will fire me? Oh my God, what am I going to do if I lose my job? I cannot afford that, I have so many bills to pay..."*). You see how it can quickly derail.

If it happens only once in a while, it is not fun, but it is not dangerous either. The problem is when you are constantly under the pressure of stress and anxiety. It can have devastating effects on the long term: insomnia, loss of appetite, illnesses, bad mood, isolation, burnout, depression and, in the worst-case scenario, it can lead to suicide cause a person is just unable to cope with the pain anymore. And these are just a few examples. Scary, huh?

But let's fear not. Solutions exist and can easily be used. Let's examine them together.

30 ways

BODY

Stress and anxiety are having a toll on your body. You probably don't feel it all the time, in fact maybe none of the time, but it's there. And the long-term effects can be perilous. Stress and anxiety produce a hormone called cortisol. It is not damageable in normal concentration, i.e. if your stress and anxiety calm down after the "threat" has passed. But when you constantly feel there is something stressful in your environment, that hormone stays in your system, and that's when problems start.

Overexposure to cortisol can disturb your body's functions. This puts you at increased risk of numerous health problems, including: digestive problems, weight gain, high blood pressure, heart disease, etc. How can a person prevent that?

Stretching and exercise

A good way to attack the problem is to start being more active. By doing so, your body produces endorphins, which are basically feel-good hormones.

If you weren't active in the last months or years, please begin slowly. Your body is not a machine; you need to give it time to adjust. Start with some gentle stretching which will help you gain more flexibility. After a couple of days of stretching, move on to something a little more challenging but still gentle to your body. No need to go overboard here. You can walk 20-30 minutes a day, do some swimming or go cycling for a bit. Do that for a couple more days/weeks in combination with the stretching.

Gradually, you will be able to do more energetic activities, if you want to. Aerobics, kick-boxing, running... you choose. If you prefer a more gentle activity, like yoga, it is perfectly fine too. You don't need to put your body through torture, you just need to move more.

I recommend that you continue to stretch regularly (daily, if possible) even though you are also doing a sport. It will give your body a chance to get rid of some tension and will also energize you, especially if you do it in the morning. As for the exercise, 30 minutes, three times a week is an absolute minimum. But if you can insert some daily exercise in your routine, that would be ideal and would benefit you the most.

Sleep

Sleep is one of the most important things to consider when trying to keep your stress and anxiety at bay. It's also one of the first things that suffer from S/A. You go to bed at night and start to think about the million things that you do not control in your life which begins a vortex of unwanted thoughts and negative feelings that keep you awake. Does that sound familiar? I bet it does.

So now, let me ask you a question. How do you go to bed every night? Do you just go to bed? Without any preparation? Well, maybe that is part of the problem. You are not giving your body any buffer between "awake and active" and "sleeping".

It is important to have a routine before going to bed to let your body know that it's time to relax and prepare to sleep. As for the length of the buffer period, it depends on each individual. I personally need almost an hour. But you could need only ten minutes. You have to try various scenarios to see what works best for you.

As an example, a good routine could be something like this:

1. Brush your teeth;
2. Put on your PJ so you are comfortable;
3. Do some gentle stretching to get rid of the tension of the day;
4. Do some breathing exercises to calm you down even further;
5. Then, go to bed.

After a couple of days, your body will begin to understand that when you start the routine, it is time to let go and put itself in sleep mode.

If you are suffering from insomnia from time to time – which can happen to anybody in a stressful period – do not roll endlessly on your mattress while fixating on the clock ticking by the hours. That is the worst thing you could do. Instead, get up and do a quiet activity for a couple of minutes to change your mindset. Something like a puzzle or reading. Do not look at the clock. When you feel your eyelids growing heavier, then go to bed. Repeat this as many times as necessary. You will eventually fall asleep, and your brain will not have the chance to establish a connexion between lying on the bed and being hopelessly awake.

Eat healthily and drink a lot

Let's put it this way: if you feed your body with crap, you will feel like crap. Simple equation. Your body is your first home, one you cannot escape or sell if it doesn't fit anymore. You are stuck with it. So better take good care of it.

It's not exactly a question of size. It's more about feeling good in your body by giving it the good things that it needs to function properly.

I'm not saying to go bio or vegan or anything like that. In Canada, we have what is called the *Canada's Food Guide*[1]. It's a good place to start. Here is how it works. The food you eat can be divided into four groups:

1. Vegetables and Fruit
2. Grain Products
3. Milk and Alternatives
4. Meat and Alternatives

A chart shows how many food servings you should eat from each food group every day. This tool ensures that you get everything that is necessary to your body.

Be careful with portions. Don't eat too much. Eat slowly as it will give the satiety signal time to reach your brain.

As to drinks, there is nothing better and more natural than water, of course. And knowing that up to 60% of the

---

[1] http://www.hc-sc.gc.ca/fn-an/food-guide-aliment/index-eng.php

human body consist of water, it could be a good idea to drink a lot of it. But there are also some healthy alternatives if you are not a big fan of water: milk, juices, herbal tea. You should drink at least eight 8-ounce glasses of water or other fluid every day. Avoid coffee and energy drinks as much as possible since they are full of caffeine. Go easy on alcohols too.

Be gentle with your body

Your body goes through a lot daily. It's being shaken in the subway, shoved in the various crowds that we engaged in, walked in high heels (for the ladies), forced to do repetitive movements over and over, assaulted by dust and chemicals of all kinds... For God's sake, give it a break once in a while!

Allow yourself to do something that feels good for your body as often as you can. It doesn't need to be complicated. A long steamy shower to relax your muscles, a bubble bath just for the fun of it or wearing comfy clothes and slippers when you're at home. If you have the money, treat yourself to a professional massage, you won't regret it. If it's not an option, ask your partner or a close friend to give you a massage in exchange for something you both decide on (a meal, another massage...).

The way that you choose does not matter. The important thing is that it gives your body pleasure. Help it to remember that it can relax from time to time.

Sex

Yes, sex. S.E.X. Sex. Sweaty, dirty, mind-blowing sex. Nothing best to take your mind off your problems than an orgasm. Seriously, how could you think about what is stressing or bothering you when your body is feeling almost liquid with pleasure and release? It is impossible.

Reacquaint yourself with sex just for the pleasure of it. Enjoy having sex with your partner. Don't just do it under the covers, in 10 minutes and then fall fast asleep. Savor it. Take your time. Swim in all those delicious sensations that are rolling through your body. Explore what feels good, what doesn't. For you and for your partner. Immerse yourselves in a bubble that only the two of you have access to.

Do not hesitate to open up to your partner about what you want, what you would like him/her do to you. If you always had a craving for something but never got the courage to try it, do it. I always had a recurring kind of fantasies when it came to the bedroom but were too scared of admitting them for a long time. After a depression and a lot of work on myself, I finally gathered up the nerve to talk about it with my husband. I was so scared he was going to feel inadequate. But to my surprise, he took it very well and also confesses to having similar fantasies. So we introduced some new practices in the bedroom, and both enjoyed our sex lives much more since then.

Sex is often relegated to the background. We'll get to it if we have some spare time. It's a mistake. Sex is something we should put on our priority list.

If you are single at the time and cannot or do not want to find somebody to have sex with, it is not a problem. Have sex with yourself. Masturbation does not have to be a taboo anymore. Self-pleasuring can also be damn good. Enjoy your body and all the wonderful sensations it can bring you. Don't be afraid, do it.

Breathe

It can sound obvious or even stupid to tell you to breathe, but it's not. When I started to do some work on myself, I realized that I stopped breathing every time something stressful came my way. I did not do it on purpose; it was a reflex, entirely automatic. So I started doing some breathing exercises, and it was very tough at the beginning. I was used to breathing superficially (only my chest was going through the motion). But the breathing exercises were designed to teach me how to breathe deeply (with my abdomen involved). I had to force myself because it wasn't natural for me. I had breathed superficially for years. But I am very glad I persisted cause it got easier with each day and I noted some benefits along the way: I was more focused, had more energy and was calmer when something unexpected happened.

I also discovered a fun app to help me with my breathing exercises. It's called *Breathing Zone*. If you have a smartphone, I encourage you to try this app. It's fun, and you can personalize it the way you want. For example, you can have a guiding voice that says "Breath in, Breath out" as you do so, or you can choose to replace the voice by a calming sound. I use the ocean waves because it reminds me of my place of birth, and it helps me calm down.

You can also combine your breathing exercises with relaxation or meditation. There are a lot of relaxing and meditating methods available. Search online, and you will find plenty. There are many tutorials on *YouTube* or apps for your smartphone. You can also decide to try a group class. Explore and find the right way for you.

MIND

Always being under pressure with S/A is also damaging for your mind and can lead to a variety of complications: elevated risk of developing mental illnesses, difficulty concentrating, depression, confusion, etc. You don't want that in your life, believe me. Here are six ways to protect your mind against stress and anxiety.

Medication

This one could be difficult to swallow, I know. But in some cases, it could be necessary. When I suffered from depression back in 2013, the doctor prescribed to me a pill named *Cymbalta*. It was the best choice for me because, as well as having a positive effect on my depression and anxiety symptoms, it was also benefiting me greatly regarding my fibromyalgia symptoms. A super-charged 3-in-1 combo pill.

There are a lot of other pills on the market, and no one works the same way as the other. That's why a good doctor is essential to advise you as to which option has the best chance of working for you.

Taking medication can be pretty scary. You could feel like a failure for not being able to conquer your demons all by yourself. You could also worry about the side-effects of taking drugs. But those thoughts serve nothing except your anxiety that feast on them. What does it matter if you need a little help to get you started on the right path? Is that utterly wrong? Does that make you less of a good person? No. Of course, it doesn't.

If you feel like there is no light in sight, like you are searching for air desperately but only end up suffocating more, if you have panic attacks, medication could be the first step to help you get out of this vicious circle. By calming your overactive thoughts, you will be able to take a step back from the anxiety and start to make gradual changes in your life so that the anxiety doesn't control you anymore.

Recognize the cycle of anxiety

I said it before, and I'll say it again: anxiety is a vicious cycle. Learning to understand its maneuvers can help you gain some control back. It usually starts with a trigger. This trigger is something that you fear, no matter how big or small it is. The trigger provokes unpleasant thoughts which feed bad feelings which bring compulsive behaviors. Those behaviors incite another flood of unpleasant thoughts, and the cycle goes on and on. Here is an example:

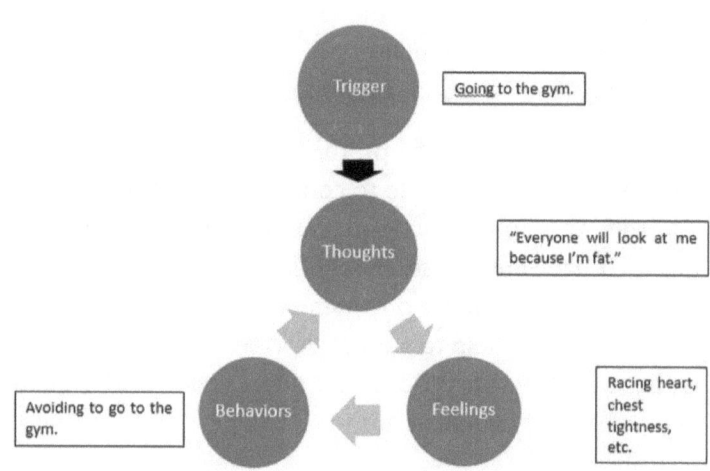

When you are stuck in the anxiety cycle, you don't even have to face the trigger: simply thinking about the trigger will start all the process. And since the cycle is unending, you can quickly become paralyzed by it. But when you know how the cycle works, you can stop it. It's not easy, but it's doable. Your power resides between the trigger and the thoughts. You must stop those thoughts any way you can. Do some physical activity, go outside, watch a movie, read a book... Anything that can distract you from your negative thoughts and that will occupy your brain with something else. You can also modify your thoughts (see next section). In the beginning, it will be hard. Your unpleasant thoughts will try to push past the distractions and invade your brain. But with perseverance, you will be able to do it more often, and it will last longer.

Modify your thoughts

This section can complement the previous one (*Recognize the cycle of anxiety*). Thoughts, especially negative ones, are the enemy. It's not easy to fight an invisible enemy that lives inside you but it's possible and with practice, it becomes easier.

When you realize that you have a negative thought, immediately replace it by a positive one. Example: if you realize you are thinking "I'm so scared about this situation," scratch that and start to tell yourself "I am strong enough to face this situation." The negative thought will not go away just like that, of course. It will try the pass through any crack it can identify and regain control back. But if you consciously decide to replace this bad thought with a positive one *every damn time* it shows up in your mind, it will eventually appear less and less and be permanently replaced by the positive one.

Since you are reading this, you are probably very familiar with anxiety and have a lot of negative thoughts in your mind. So in the beginning, you will have the impression of always blocking bad thoughts and you may feel overwhelmed by the magnitude of it and thinking that it's a lost cause and that you will never win this. But mark my word, perseverance is the key and yes, it will work.

See a therapist

There are probably reasons why you are stuck in this S/A cycle. A therapist could help you find them and resolve them.

Choosing a therapist can be tricky. You need to find someone which you are at ease with, which you will not hesitate to share you deepest thoughts with. But you also need someone who will challenge you by asking the right questions, which means questions that will help you to dig through your thoughts and feeling and find the answers that you need to move forward.

That being said, I believe that consulting a therapist can only last for so long. It cannot become a permanent crutch. If that is the case, you are not moving forward. A therapist should help you to get through a time of need and give you the tools you need to continue on your own afterward. If another tough time presents itself a couple of months or years later, you can always contact her/him at that particular time, though.

A great therapist should be like a mirror and help you to know yourself better.

Take a break from technology

Chances are you would probably have a panic attack if you lose your smartphone. I bet your whole life is in it: all your contacts, your emails, your games, your social media accounts, your schedule, your banking information, your photos, etc. While it is nice to have everything on one device, it can also become an addiction if you always need to use it.

In 2015, daily time spent by users on their smartphone was almost 3 hours[2]. When adding daily time spent in front of a screen (smartphone, laptop, TV, etc.), it climbs to almost 10 hours! That's incredible. Technology submerges us, and we don't even realize it no more because it's become the norm. It is now a vital need to retrace any information on a right here, right now basis.

But this comes at a price: isolation (you connect with people only by text or social medias and don't see them face to face as often as you used to), sleep disturbance (the artificial light from TV and computer screens affects our melatonin production and throws off circadian rhythms which prevents deep and restorative sleep), obesity (cause you move less), constant distraction (your phone or computer is always buzzing or beeping to signal a new message or email) and many more negative side effects.

---

[2]   http://www.smartinsights.com/mobile-marketing/mobile-marketing-analytics/mobile-marketing-statistics/

I'm not going to tell you to stop using all your devices altogether. That would not be realistic. We live in a modern society. But I am going to encourage you to put some distance between you and technology. Stop the many notifications on your phone, so it's not buzzing/beeping all the time. Do not stop what you're doing every time an email pops in; reserve a specific time to check that. Use social medias a little less: nobody cares if you ate a sandwich or soup at lunch. Instead of playing games on your phone while in the subway, bring a good book and read. Try to detach yourself from all of that and think of technology as a tool, not a vital need.

Take your mind off things

If you consistently focus your attention on your problems, on your stress and your anxiety, you will go nuts. Period. Just like your body needs a break once in a while, your brain does too. Maybe even more cause the majority of our struggles are internal.

Take your mind off what is bothering you by focusing on something else. Try a new hobby, take a class of some sort, go out with friends. Read a book, do your laundry, pay your bills. Anything.

As we saw before, anxiety feeds on your negative thoughts and emotions. So cut it out. Don't give it anything to grow upon. Mentally shake yourself and choose to place your focus on something else, preferably something fun cause it will work even better.

HEART

A person under the constant weight of S/A can only hide it for so long. Inevitably, revealing signs are going to appear: irritability, edginess, overreaction to little annoyances, isolation, frequent crying episodes, and much more. You feel like you are all alone in this storm and that no one can understand what you're going through. But here are some ways to mend your wounded heart.

Talk to a friend

When we are stuck within the S/A cycle, we often draw ourselves from the people around us. We are so scared of being judged by others, even the ones that love us unconditionally, that we keep everything that's bothering us bottled up inside. I did that for countless years.

When I cracked, it wasn't pretty. It all came out like a flood one afternoon with one of my friends. To my total disbelief, I didn't feel bad for sharing my ugliest thoughts and didn't feel judged by this friend. On the contrary, he made me feel loved, secured and even got a laugh or two out of me, which dedramatized the situation.

I felt better after emptying my emotional bag. It didn't magically solve all my problems, but it allowed me to release some pressure off.

It's important to have loyal friends like that, friends you can count on, friends who will listen to your story, to your pain, and try to make you feel better. If you have a friend like that in your entourage, do not hesitate to confide in her/him. She/he could be of great help.

Adopt an animal

Having another living creature to focus on except yourself can do you a lot of good. The all-time winner in this category is the dog. You simply cannot obsess over everything in your head when your dog is demanding to go outside to do his business. It's relentless. It will follow you everywhere in the house, bark, cry, jump on you, whatever is necessary to make you understand that you must take it outside NOW.

Of course, if you hate dogs, don't bring one into your home. A lot of animals can occupy you just as well: a cat, a rabbit, a bird... go with your heart on this one. Cause needless to say that an animal needs a lot of care and can live up to 20 years, so it's a long-term commitment.

But this little or big ball of fur (or feathers, or...) will bring you so much joy. And it will always love you and be here for you, no matter how crappy you feel or whatever you confess. It will always look at you with the same adoring eyes.

Animals are also very funny from time to time. It will do the funniest faces, run after its tale or try to catch a bug or something that will make you erupt into laughter. Live those little moments to the fullest. They are precious and will mend your heart.

Some animals are also very affectionate. They will kiss (read: LICK!) you, cuddle up with you and be near you all the time. After all, you are the center of their world.

If you decide to go that way, please think it through carefully, though. Animals are living creatures with real feelings and needs. Once you adopt one, it is not ok to abandon it at the first problem. So better ask yourself a bunch of questions before hands. Are you allergic to pets? Do you have a lot of energy or are you more a stay-at-home kind of gal? Do you live in a tiny apartment or do you own a house? Do you have a backyard and if so, is it fenced? How much money will you be able to spend on your pet on a monthly basis? And so on... Go on the Internet and Google "Questions to ask before adopting a pet" and you will find a ton of good sites to help you evaluate all the necessary aspects.

If after weighting the pros and cons, you decide that this is something for you, I personally recommend that you visit an animal shelter near you and that you adopt a pet over there. Not only will you save two lives (the pet that you adopt and the one that will be able to take the vacant spot at the shelter) but you can almost be sure that this animal was well-treated for its time at the shelter. Which unfortunately cannot always be said of some pure breeders who are only there to make a quick buck.

Volunteer

Helping others is one of the best ways to focus on something else than yourself + to feel good about yourself. You can volunteer in so many ways; I'm sure you can find something that will please you. You can do administrative work, read to the elderly, socialize animals, ask people to make donations to an association, become a "big sister" or "big brother" to a kid in need, organize a show, serve food to homeless people, etc. There are almost no limits.

Do a quick research on the Internet or read your local newspaper. A lot of organizations are searching for volunteers. And most of the time, you need no previous experience but just a strong will to learn and a positive attitude. You can start slowly, like 3 hours a week, and increase gradually if you feel like it and have the time to do so.

Go for something that sparks a little light in you when you think about it. We all have causes close to our heart. Start there.

Maybe you wanted to volunteer for a while but never made the move because you were scared that you would see too many sad things and that would be too much for you. As I understand the premise, I can assure you that in reality, it is not how it works. Of course, you will see sad things once in a while, and that is part of the whole volunteering experience. But the joy and the feeling of self-contentment that will be with you every time you help someone in need will take the first place in your heart and will soothe the rest.

I volunteer with cats at the SPCA of my region. I deal mostly with the tough cases: shy ones, scared ones, aggressive ones... We have a protocol to respect to socialize those difficult cats and make them understand that humans can be good for them. Sometimes, it works very fast, and a cat can become friendly in a couple of hours. But other days, we have cats that take weeks, even months, to rehabilitate. But when it finally works and they get adopted by a good family, it is the most gratifying thing ever.

Positive affirmations

This one is part of the "fake it 'til you make it" category. I was pretty doubtful when I tried this at first, but it really works. If you are 100% committed, it will do wonders for you too. The basis is simple. You start with the phrase "I am ..." and then you insert the word of your choice. For example, you could say "I am happy." Choose a quality that you would like to have or a trait of personality that you would like to put emphasis on and repeat it like a mantra. Everyday. At any chance you can get.

You can choose to focus on a single item or make it a combo. When I started, I was doing the combo thing and saying to myself all the time "I am energetic, strong, confident and positive." At the time, it was what I needed to remind myself of. Over the years, I changed the words and the number of words to provide me with what I needed most when I needed it.

You will probably – no, scratch that – you will *totally* feel silly doing this at first. But don't dwell on that and just do it, you'll thank me later. You can start by just thinking it in your head the first days. But eventually, as you grow accustomed to the words, I encourage you to say them out loud. That will multiply their power.

Why does this work? How can something so simple help you feel and act according to those words that you are saying every day? Is it faith? Magic? Placebo effect? Not at all. It is based on one simple fact: your brain accepts everything that you are saying as true and start to think and act accordingly. It is not capable of discerning what is true of what is false. So if you thought and even heard all your life that you were a failure, that you were ugly or anything right up that alley, your brain just accepted that and started to act like it was really a fact.

Knowing that, you can consciously alter how your brain is wired by saying positive affirmations about yourself on a daily basis. Consistency is the key here. The more you say it, the more your brain will accept it and the more you'll start to feel free to be who you truly are.

Sensory delight

When you want to feel better, immerse your senses in bliss. It can be anything that soothes you or else, motivates you. For example:

Soothing: Waves sounds on the beach.

Motivating: Pop music to dance along while doing your weekly house cleaning.

Find what appeals to you, what can transport you elsewhere in a second. A lot of those can be related to happy childhood memories: food that your mom used to cook, an old blanket that felt so soft against your skin, and old melody that your grandma sang to you... Whatever it is, it must trigger calm or joy in you. When you identify these things, do not hesitate to reproduce them consciously to trigger that ecstasy feeling that they always bring.

Assume yourself

You are a unique individual with your own values, likes, dislikes, and opinions. Be proud of who you are, don't be ashamed. Even if you are against the current, it is entirely okay to be YOU with all that entails. If you try to conceal your real identity or personality, that will cause problems in other areas of your life.

I am bisexual. And I had a lot of difficulties accepting that. The main reason is that I was making a wrong association when I thought about that. For me, being bisexual equaled ending my relationship with my husband. I thought if I come out, he would not be okay with that and leave me. I struggled with that fear for a few years. But when I suffered from depression in 2013, I decided that I finally wanted to be true to myself, that it was time to let the real me shine. So I told my husband and expected to worst...

He did not make a triple joy spin, but he did not pack his luggage either. He was mostly worried: does that meant that I wanted to leave him and sleep with women? I was then able to reassure him: I did not want to leave him, I was still very in love with him, and even though I had a desire for women, I did not want to sleep with anybody (male or female) that wasn't him. After that, we understood each other better, and our relationship continued to grow. I am still with him to this day.

I was so relieved that it went well, but that was only the beginning. I hadn't realized that hiding this part of me was affecting me in other spheres of my life. I always thought I was ugly before that. After spitting out my big secret, I was finally able to see the beauty in me. I always had some inhibitions in the bedroom. With that burden off my mind, my inhibitions just disappeared. I also felt happier a lot of the time and more myself. I was finally comfortable in my skin.

This is why I encourage you to assume yourself, to embrace everything that makes you unique and YOU.

SOUL

S/A is so much of a burden, it can destroy a lot of things in its wake, leaving you with these not-so-fun symptoms: feeling overwhelmed, difficulty in making decisions, lack of motivation, reduced productivity, etc. What can you do to avoid that?

Simplify your life

It seems that the motto of a lot of people these days could be: why keeping it simple when you can have it complicated? And this is a total non-sense. Why do we feel the need to overwhelm us with everything? And I mean EVERYTHING. We want to do everything, we want to have everything, we want to know everything. News flash, guys: it's impossible. You will only exhaust yourself in trying to do so.

I think this is where we need to remind ourselves that life is about making choices. You want to save up for an all-inclusive vacation in Mexico, well you will have to dial down on dining at the restaurant 5 (five) times a week. You want to do volunteer work; well you probably won't have the time to go back to school like you wanted. You want to work and have kids, well you should consider working part-time only or hiring someone to help you with domestic chores.

You cannot have everything in life. You need to prioritize what is most important to you and act accordingly. If not, you will end up missing something eventually: money, energy or time. This can't work in the long run.

I know sometimes making choices can be scary because we don't want to miss out on anything. But it is not a crime to choose to focus on something specific for a while. You can always change your mind in the future if you want to. Nothing is carved in stone. You can make a change if a situation does not please you.

Adjust your standards

Do you feel the need for perfection? In everything that you say and do? That's a common problem in anxious people. I sincerely used to believe that I had to be at my best all the time to have the love and respect from others in my life. That meant: always be well-dressed, be nice to everybody, having perfect scores in class, only be remarked for my excellent work at my job, etc. It was EXHAUSTING. I have no word for it. It's like a constant battle to be the best in all the facets of your life, never letting your guard down in any situation or for anybody.

I hit my first wall, so to speak, when I was 23. I had to take the driving test *three times* before passing it. I was beside myself with disbelief. What was wrong with me all of a sudden? Why couldn't I get it the first time? What would everyone think of me?? I was such a **loser**! And then what happened? Absolutely nothing. Nobody was shocked that I didn't have it the first time. Nobody thought I was less of a good person because of it. It was the beginning of a new phase for me.

Of course, I did not go from Miss-crazy-perfection to Miss-Does-Not-Give-A-Damn in a day. But with time, I understood that I did not need to be perfect to be loved, that allowing myself to be less than perfect did not diminish my worth.

Keep things in perspective

This one goes hand-in-hand with the previous one (*Adjust your standards*). We, anxious people, have a lot of difficulties to be objective, especially when we are involved in the situation. Everything always seems so damn precarious, like the end of the world could happen for any reason. We missed our bus and are going to be late for work? End of the world. We dropped something on our pants, and it's made a teeny tiny stain? End of the world. Did we forget to call somebody? End of the world. It is always the end of the world.

But this is just ridiculous. Nothing is the end the world. Not even losing our job or breaking up with the one we love. It is not because something unpleasant happens to us that the Earth will stop turning. In fact, it's pretty self-involved to think that way. We are over 7 billion people on this planet. And I can assure you that while you are living an embarrassing or unpleasant moment, there are *at least* 1 billion people who are living something way worse at the same time. So please, let's put things in perspective.

Let's revisit the examples in the first paragraph. You missed your bus and are going to be late for work? Call your boss to advise her/him that you'll be late. You dropped something on your pants, and it's made a teeny tiny stain? You'll wash that at home and in the meantime, no one cares. Did you forget to call somebody? Call this person and apologize. See how there is always a simple solution?

Let go

So something happened, and it did not go the way you expected or wanted? So what? Is obsessing about it will change anything? No. So let it go. The past is the past, and you cannot change it in any way. Choose to see the situation as a learning experience instead, and then move on.

Now and then, you will also be confronted by a situation that you would like to handle differently, but it will not be possible. You can stand your ground and make a scene and try to bring back the power in your hands. But if it's not that important, you can also choose to let it go. That does not make you a push-over. You simply choose to put your energy elsewhere that is more important to you.

For example: let's say that you moved in with your new boyfriend. He wants to paint the bedroom in gray, and you want it yellow. If the bedroom is the most important room in the house for you, you could choose to argue with your boyfriend. But if you realize that the most significant place for you is rather the kitchen, you could decide to let your boyfriend "win" this one if he accepts to let you choose the color in the kitchen instead. That would be a great compromise, and you would not have to put energy in an argument when you don't want to.

The main thing to keep from all of this is: you are the only one to decide where you want to put your energy.

Know your limits and learn to say "no."

This section is the complement of the previous one (*Let go*). While it is important to let go of the less important stuff, you don't want to let go of everything and always agreeing with what others say. If you do that, people will take advantage of you. That is why you must know your limits and learn to say "no" when it is necessary.

Like I said before, you need to choose where you want to put your energy. If you're always saying yes when someone suggests something or asks you to do something, you will eventually be missing time, money or energy. Do not be uncomfortable refusing an invitation, for example. You have the right to be busy elsewhere or just wanting a calm evening at home for a change. No need to justify yourself. Do not feel bad for not helping a friend to move. You could have previous plans or not being in a shape good enough to lift heavy furniture for an entire day. You could also offer to help in another way, like cooking two or three meals to give your moving friend a chance to eat well until he has time to go to the grocery in his new neighborhood.

Think outside of the box.

Be in nature

Do not just go outside, especially in you live in the city. Go out and be in nature. Walk in a forest or a field or flowers, lay on the beach and listen to the waves, or go hiking on a mountain. Being in contact with nature is important. We are all so caught up in busy lives, going from home to work and back and forth, taking care of the house and the children, having a social life, that we rarely make time to reconnect with nature. But it is part of us, and we are part of it.

It is also beneficial to be reminded of our smallness in the face of nature. Personally, I love to watch the stars in the sky at night. I feel so little, and it humbles me. It is also really pretty and kind of magical to see all those little lights sparkling above me.

Nature is essential to our survival, and we should learn to be thankful for that. We can breathe because of the trees that release oxygen into the atmosphere, we can eat because of the food (animal or vegetal) that nature provides us, we can drink because of the pure water that nature shares with us. And humans are only a kind of particularly developed animal. So we are connected to nature, and we need it to continue to live. Might as well spend some time in it and learn to respect and love it.

ACTION

The last area of which you can have an impact on is your actions. S/A can lead to a wide series of negative behaviors like nervous habits, Obsessive Compulsive Disorder (OCD), increased alcohol or drug use, impulse buying, etc. Before you get there or to replace those negative behaviors, you can try these few ideas.

Smile

This one is also part of the "fake it 'til you make it" category. Yes, you will feel stupid when you do smile but don't want to for the first time. But did you know this: a smile can improve your mood and reduce your stress level. Yep, yep. Your brain immediately releases endorphins when you smile, even if it is a forced smile. Your brain does not see the difference between a real smile and a fake one. Amazing, huh?

Smiling is also contagious. Try this little exercise for a week and you'll see what I'm talking about: smile to at least five strangers every day. The vast majority of these people will smile back to you – maybe some will even come and talk to you because when you smile, you look approachable! – and they are most likely to be in a good mood after that and also smile to other strangers.

A smile also makes you look younger and more attractive. Hey, that's a plus! So if you don't have time to put your makeup on one morning, try smiling the rest of the day, that should do the trick.

Studies have as well demonstrated that smiling helps you gain someone else's trust. Probably because the brain unconsciously thinks that a happy person looks less threatening than a frowning one.

So there are a lot of good reasons to smile more, for you and the ones around you. And since it's free, do not hesitate to spread your smiles at anytime, anywhere.

Get out of the house

Is there anything more depressing than looking at the same four walls while rehashing some negative thoughts over and over again? I don't think so. While it can be good to have some quiet time at home, if you stay there because you are more in a hiding mood, that is not the solution. In fact, it will probably leave you more depressed in the end.

In this state, it would be more beneficial for you to go out and do something. Invite a friend to brunch at your favorite restaurant, go to the movies and watch a comedy, take the dog for a walk, or take a bike ride. No need to be out for the entire day but just enough to change your mood (I would say at least thirty minutes). If you are an introverted person, try to make that a daily habit. It will do you good to shake things up a little and change your routine.

Manage your time/prepare

S/A can also come from a lack a time management or preparation. So I suggest that you look into that. Do you manage your time at all or do you just go with the flow? As an example, do you go to the groceries one day and to the pharmacy another day, even though they are relatively close to one another? If you'd go to both places in the same outing, you could save driving time and free one more evening that given week. Try to regroup what can be done at the same time.

If you are slow in the morning and always running late, why don't you prepare every possible thing the night before? Make your lunch, choose your outfit, place everything you might need (purse, keys, wallet, scarf...) close to the door, so you don't have to search for them when the morning comes.

When you have an exam in school or a presentation at work, allow yourself enough time ahead to revise or practice what you need to know for the big day.

Put little notes on the fridge or use your smartphone so you don't forget what's important. Ask help from your family or friends if it's possible. For example: if you do the dishes while your partner vacuums the place, you could both relax together afterward. That is not rocket science.

Make a list

I love making lists. I even bought a book on that subject! People think I'm a bit of a freak but who cares? It really helps me put order in my head. Thoughts are usually flying in my mind, but when I order them on paper in a neat list, it soothes me and I can sort through them without panicking.

You can make lists for anything. From groceries to clothes you need to buy to places you want to visit before you die, there is absolutely no limit. It can be very useful for the practical stuff (ex.: items you need to bring with you on vacation), but it can also be inspirational (ex.: languages you want to learn).

It is also most helpful when making a hard decision. You then make a "pros/cons list" for a given situation. I always do that when I'm torn, and it helps me to visualize the whole situation resumed on one sheet of paper.

When I feel stressed out (thankfully it happens less and less these days), I also write down a stress list. I write everything that stresses me and then ranks each item from one to ten (ten being the highest stressor possible). I can then work through that list to eliminate some sources of stress. I don't always work the same way. Sometimes I begin with what stresses me the most cause, obviously, I want to get rid of that. But sometimes I start with some items that stress me less so I can concentrate more about finding a solution to what stresses me the most afterward. Do what feels natural at the moment, do not question yourself endlessly.

Clean, declutter, organize

If you are like me, the chances are that your surroundings at home or work reflect how you truly feel inside. When I feel good, my house is usually clean and decluttered. But when a million thoughts race through my head and I don't know where to begin to put some order in them, my house looks like a mess. But what is interesting is that I noticed over time that the reverse could also apply. When I bring order in my house, it unconsciously helps me to bring order to my mind too.

I'm not a hoarder or anything approaching that, but I still like to keep things "just in case". But almost every time I do that, I clutter my house with something unnecessary. That's why about four times a year (at each season), I do a big declutter day (or weekend). I then rummage through the entire house and ask myself if I really *need* that object. I usually fill up two or three big bags for charity and as much are going in the trash. I never regretted anything I got rid of.

It is also important to organize your space the most efficiently possible so you can easily find or access what you need, which results in less stress. Put all the books in bookshelves, store all your photos at the same place, hang all your scarves on hooks, install a bowl near the door to deposit your keys in, regroup all cleaning products under the sink. You get the idea.

If you have the money to do so, hire someone to do a weekly cleaning of the house. Or reserve a specific moment in your schedule to do it yourself. You will function way more efficiently and happily in a clean environment.

Exposition

Finally, it is possible to reduce your stress and anxiety to a given situation by slowly exposing yourself to it. *Slowly* being the key word here. You don't want to go too fast and then create a trauma because that would be tough to get over that.

For example, in my early twenties, I was scared of going in elevators. It was not a rational fear, nothing bad ever happened to me in one. But I was scared no matter what. I then got a job at the fifth floor of a building. Since my cardio was not that good, taking the elevator was a more attractive option all of a sudden. But I still feared it. So I went gradually. I started by taking the elevator when there were people inside cause I thought that was less scary (at least, if I were to be stuck in it, I wouldn't be alone). Then I tried going in alone but focusing my attention on something else (a book, music on my mp3 player, anything). And one day, I finally realized that I was not scared anymore. I even got stuck in an elevator once and did not flinch at all. I was very proud of myself.

You can accomplish that too. Whether it's a dog phobia or fear of talking in public, you can overcome anything you put your mind to. If your fear is more on the panic side, I recommend that you enroll a professional to help you, though. You don't have to go through this all alone, and it's ok if you progress very slowly. The important thing is that you continue to try.

Conclusion

Getting rid of your stress and anxiety and gaining control back over your life cannot be done in one day with just one magical remedy. It takes time, dedication, perseverance and a combination of several ways described in this book. But it's a small price to pay to finally be happy in your skin.